I0774066

Obesity Myths Busted
The Real Secrets to Shedding Pounds

Table of Contents:

Chapter 1
The Biggest Myths About Obesity and Why They're Wrong

Are you tired of the endless cycle of diets and exercise routines that promise weight loss but deliver little to no results? It's time to uncover the truth behind obesity and weight loss – the real secrets that will help you shed those stubborn pounds for good. Let's break free from the common misconceptions that have been holding us back. It's time to challenge the myths that have been ingrained in our minds for far too long. By understanding the truth, we can finally take the right steps towards achieving lasting and sustainable weight loss. Conventional wisdom often leads us astray when it comes to dieting and weight management. We've been told to simply eat less and move more, but the reality is far more complex. There are hidden factors at play, influencing our weight in ways we may not have considered before. In this book, we delve deep into the science behind weight gain and obesity. We explore the role of metabolism, hormones, and genetics in shaping our bodies and influencing our weight. By understanding these factors, we can tailor our approach to weight loss in a way that works best for us as individuals. Say goodbye to one-size-fits-all solutions and welcome a personalized plan that truly fits your lifestyle and needs. It's time to take control of your health and well-being, armed with the knowledge and tools to make a real difference in your life. With practical advice, easy-to-follow strategies, and inspiring success stories, this book is your roadmap to a healthier, happier you. Let's debunk the myths, embrace the truth, and start our journey towards a transformed and empowered self.

Chapter 2
Effective, Sustainable Weight Loss Techniques

Are you tired of feeling like you're trapped in a cycle of failed diets and unfulfilled fitness goals? It's time to break free from the shackles of misinformation and discover the real secrets to shedding those stubborn pounds for good. In this chapter, we will delve into the core principles of effective and sustainable weight loss techniques that have been proven to deliver long-lasting results. No more quick fixes or temporary solutions – it's time to embrace a holistic approach to your health and well-being. One of the key insights we will explore is the importance of debunking common myths surrounding obesity and weight loss. By understanding the truth behind these misconceptions, you can pave the way for a more informed and successful weight loss journey. Furthermore, we will uncover the role of metabolism, hormones, and genetics in the complex landscape of weight management. By gaining a deeper understanding of these factors, you can tailor your approach to weight loss to suit your unique biological makeup and personal needs. But knowledge alone is not enough – practical advice and easy-to-follow strategies are essential for translating theory into tangible results. From setting realistic goals to implementing sustainable lifestyle changes, this chapter will equip you with the tools you need to take charge of your health and transform your body. And let's not forget the power of motivation and inspiration. Throughout this chapter, you will encounter uplifting success stories that demonstrate the real-life impact of effective weight loss techniques. These stories serve as a reminder that lasting change is not only possible but within your reach. So, say goodbye to the cycle of frustration and hello to a brighter, healthier future. By embracing the principles outlined in this chapter, you will embark on a transformative journey towards a happier, more confident you. It's time to reclaim your health and well-being – are you ready to take the first step towards a better tomorrow?

Chapter 3
The Role of Metabolism, Hormones, and Genetics in Weight Management

Are you tired of feeling defeated by the number on the scale? Have you tried countless diets and exercise routines only to be left disappointed and discouraged? It's time to shift your focus from quick fixes to understanding the true factors at play when it comes to weight management. In the journey towards shedding pounds and achieving a healthier lifestyle, it's crucial to debunk the common misconceptions surrounding obesity. By unraveling the myths that have been ingrained in our minds for so long, we can pave the way for real, sustainable change. One of the key elements in this process is recognizing the intricate interplay between metabolism, hormones, and genetics. These factors are not to be underestimated; they hold the key to unlocking your body's potential for effective weight management. Metabolism, often seen as the body's internal furnace, plays a vital role in determining how efficiently we burn calories. While some are blessed with a naturally speedy metabolism, others may have a slower rate that makes weight loss more challenging. Understanding your metabolic rate can help tailor your approach to diet and exercise, ensuring that you are working with your body, not against it. Hormones, the chemical messengers in our bodies, also wield significant influence over our weight. From insulin and cortisol to leptin and ghrelin, these hormones can impact our appetite, energy levels, and fat storage. By learning how to regulate these hormones through lifestyle choices and nutrition, you can create a more harmonious internal environment conducive to weight loss. Genetics, though often viewed as a predetermined factor, do not have to dictate your destiny. While it's true that certain genetic traits can influence how your body responds to food and exercise, they do not have the final say. By understanding your genetic predispositions, you can tailor your weight management approach to optimize your results. Ultimately, achieving lasting weight loss requires a holistic understanding of your body and its unique needs. By embracing the role of metabolism, hormones, and genetics in weight management, you can create a personalized plan that sets you up for success. It's time to break free from the limitations of conventional wisdom and empower yourself with the knowledge needed to transform your health and well-being.

Chapter 4
How to Develop a Personalized Plan That Fits Your Lifestyle

In the journey to overcome obesity and achieve lasting weight loss, one of the most crucial steps is developing a personalized plan that fits seamlessly into your lifestyle. This tailored approach is key to ensuring that your efforts are sustainable, effective, and ultimately successful. Creating a plan that is personalized to you involves taking into account your unique preferences, habits, schedule, and goals. By customizing your weight loss strategy, you are more likely to stay motivated and committed to the process. To begin developing your personalized plan, start by setting realistic and achievable goals. These goals should be specific, measurable, and time-bound. Whether your aim is to lose a certain amount of weight, improve your overall health, or enhance your fitness level, having clear objectives will give you a sense of direction and purpose. Next, consider your current lifestyle and identify areas where you can make positive changes. This could involve reassessing your eating habits, incorporating more physical activity into your daily routine, or prioritizing self-care and stress management. By pinpointing areas for improvement, you can gradually implement small, sustainable changes that will have a significant impact on your weight loss journey. It's essential to choose strategies that align with your preferences and personality. If you enjoy certain types of physical activity, such as dancing or hiking, incorporate these activities into your routine to make exercise more enjoyable and engaging. Likewise, if you have specific dietary preferences or restrictions, find healthy and delicious recipes that cater to your needs to ensure that you stay satisfied and nourished. Consistency is key when it comes to maintaining a personalized weight loss plan. Establishing healthy habits and routines that you can stick to in the long term will help you stay on track and avoid setbacks. Remember that progress takes time, and it's normal to encounter challenges along the way. Stay focused on your goals, stay positive, and celebrate your achievements, no matter how small they may seem. By developing a personalized plan that suits your lifestyle, preferences, and goals, you are taking a significant step towards achieving lasting weight loss and overall well-being. Embrace the journey, stay committed, and believe in your ability to transform your health and your life for the better.

Chapter 5
Understanding the Science Behind Obesity and Weight Loss

Obesity is a complex and multifaceted issue that goes far beyond just eating too much or not exercising enough. It's crucial to understand the science behind obesity and weight loss in order to effectively address and overcome this challenge. One of the biggest myths surrounding obesity is the idea that it simply boils down to willpower. Many people believe that those struggling with their weight just need to eat less and move more. While this may seem like a straightforward solution, the reality is much more nuanced. Factors such as genetics, metabolism, and hormonal imbalances play a significant role in determining an individual's weight. Some people may have a genetic predisposition to storing fat more easily, while others may have a slower metabolism that makes weight loss more challenging. Hormones, such as insulin and leptin, also play a crucial role in regulating appetite and metabolism. Understanding these underlying factors is essential for developing effective and sustainable weight loss strategies. It's not just about following the latest fad diet or workout trend; it's about creating a personalized plan that takes into account your unique biology and lifestyle. Another common misconception is that all calories are created equal. While it's true that consuming fewer calories than you burn is essential for weight loss, the quality of those calories matters just as much. Foods high in sugar, processed ingredients, and unhealthy fats can wreak havoc on your metabolism and make it harder to shed pounds. In contrast, a diet rich in whole, nutrient-dense foods can support weight loss efforts by providing essential vitamins, minerals, and antioxidants that promote overall health. Balancing macronutrients such as protein, carbohydrates, and fats is also key to optimizing metabolism and energy levels. Ultimately, the science behind obesity and weight loss is about finding a sustainable approach that works for you. It's not about quick fixes or drastic measures, but rather about making small, manageable changes that lead to long-term success. By understanding the complexities of obesity and weight loss, you can empower yourself to take control of your health and achieve lasting results. With the right knowledge and mindset, you can overcome the challenges of obesity and embark on a journey towards a healthier, happier you.

Chapter 6
Breaking Free from Fad Diets and Fitness Trends

In a world inundated with quick-fix solutions and trendy weight loss programs, it's easy to fall into the trap of fad diets and fitness trends that promise miraculous results. However, the reality is often far from what these programs claim. The key to true and lasting weight loss lies in breaking free from the cycle of chasing after the next popular diet or exercise craze and instead focusing on sustainable, evidence-based strategies. It's time to debunk the myths surrounding obesity and understand the real secrets to shedding pounds. By delving into the science behind weight loss, we can uncover the factors that truly influence our ability to reach our health goals. Rather than relying on one-size-fits-all approaches, we must recognize the individual complexities that contribute to weight management, such as metabolism, hormones, and genetics. One of the biggest misconceptions about weight loss is the idea that a drastic, restrictive diet is the only way to see results. In reality, sustainable weight loss is achieved through a balanced approach that considers both nutrition and physical activity. By developing a personalized plan that aligns with your lifestyle and preferences, you can create lasting habits that support your health journey. It's essential to shift our focus from short-term fixes to long-term wellness. Instead of viewing weight loss as a temporary goal, we must reframe our mindset to prioritize overall health and well-being. This shift in perspective empowers us to make choices that nourish our bodies and minds, leading to sustainable and meaningful results. By understanding the truth behind obesity and weight loss, we can liberate ourselves from the cycle of fad diets and fitness trends. Let go of the frustration and disappointment that often accompany quick-fix solutions, and embrace a holistic approach to health that honors your unique needs and goals. The journey to breaking free from the allure of fad diets and fitness trends starts with a commitment to self-care and a willingness to explore the proven strategies that will guide you towards lasting transformation.

Chapter 7
Empowering Yourself to Take Control of Your Health

Are you tired of feeling overwhelmed by the constant barrage of conflicting information about obesity and weight loss? Do you find yourself stuck in a cycle of trying every new diet or exercise trend only to end up right back where you started, or worse, even further from your health goals? It's time to take a step back and reevaluate the approach you're taking towards your health journey. In the journey to shed pounds and achieve a healthier lifestyle, it's essential to cut through the noise and focus on what truly matters. Let's debunk the myths that have been holding you back and discover the real secrets to sustainable weight loss and overall well-being. One of the first steps to empowering yourself is to understand the biggest misconceptions surrounding obesity. It's time to challenge the status quo and dig deeper into the root causes of weight gain. By uncovering the truth behind common myths, you can start making informed decisions that will set you on the path to success. Effective weight loss is not about quick fixes or temporary solutions. It's about implementing sustainable techniques that work for your unique body and lifestyle. By learning how to nurture your metabolism, balance your hormones, and navigate your genetic predispositions, you can develop a personalized plan that sets you up for long-term success. Taking control of your health means taking ownership of your choices. It's about recognizing that you have the power to transform your life and make lasting changes for the better. By embracing this mindset and committing to your well-being, you can break free from the cycle of frustration and disappointment. Remember, your health journey is a marathon, not a sprint. It's about making small, consistent changes that add up to significant results over time. By setting realistic goals, staying committed to your plan, and seeking support when needed, you can empower yourself to take control of your health and create the vibrant, healthy life you deserve. So, are you ready to step into your power and reclaim your health? The journey may not always be easy, but with determination, resilience, and a willingness to learn, you can achieve the transformation you've been dreaming of. Start today, and watch as you become the best version of yourself – inside and out.

Chapter 8
Inspiring Success Stories of Lasting Weight Loss

Embarking on a journey towards lasting weight loss can often feel like navigating through a maze of conflicting information and false promises. It's easy to become disheartened after trying numerous diets and exercise regimens without seeing the results you desire. But fear not, for within the pages of this book, you will find the keys to unlocking the secrets of shedding pounds for good. Let me introduce you to individuals who have walked the path you are on now. People who, like you, have faced the challenges of obesity and have emerged victorious in their quest for lasting weight loss. Their stories are not just tales of triumph but beacons of hope, guiding you towards your own success. One such inspiring story is that of Sarah, who struggled with her weight for years, trying every quick-fix solution that crossed her path. It wasn't until she shifted her focus from temporary results to long-term health that she began to see a transformation. By adopting sustainable lifestyle changes and embracing a balanced approach to nutrition and exercise, Sarah not only shed the excess pounds but also regained her confidence and vitality. Then there's John, whose battle with obesity seemed insurmountable until he discovered the power of mindset. By shifting his perspective from viewing weight loss as a punishment to seeing it as a journey of self-discovery and empowerment, John was able to break free from the cycle of yo-yo dieting and finally achieve the lasting results he had always dreamed of. These success stories, and many others like them, serve as a reminder that lasting weight loss is not just about numbers on a scale but a holistic transformation that encompasses mind, body, and spirit. By learning from those who have walked the path before you, you too can overcome the obstacles that stand in your way and embrace a healthier, happier future. So, as you read through these inspiring tales of triumph over obesity, remember that you are not alone in your journey. With perseverance, dedication, and the right guidance, you too can rewrite your story and achieve the lasting weight loss you deserve.

Chapter 9
Uncovering the Hidden Factors That Contribute to Weight Gain

In the quest to shed pounds and achieve optimal health, it's crucial to uncover the hidden factors that contribute to weight gain. While many individuals struggling with obesity may feel overwhelmed by the myriad of advice and information available, it's essential to cut through the noise and focus on the core factors that truly impact weight management. One of the most common misconceptions about weight gain is that it is solely the result of consuming too many calories and not exercising enough. While diet and physical activity certainly play a significant role, there are often underlying factors at play that can sabotage even the most well-intentioned efforts. Metabolism, for instance, is a key player in the weight management game. While some individuals may have a naturally fast metabolism that allows them to burn calories more efficiently, others may have a slower metabolism that makes weight loss more challenging. Understanding your own metabolic rate can help you tailor your approach to weight loss accordingly. Hormones also play a crucial role in weight management. Imbalances in hormones such as insulin, cortisol, and leptin can make it difficult to lose weight, even with a strict diet and exercise regimen. By addressing these hormonal imbalances through targeted lifestyle changes and, if necessary, medical intervention, individuals can unlock the key to sustainable weight loss. Genetics, too, can influence our predisposition to weight gain. While we can't change our genetic makeup, we can use this knowledge to inform our approach to weight management. By understanding our genetic tendencies and working with them rather than against them, we can create a personalized plan that is tailored to our unique needs and challenges. By delving beneath the surface and uncovering the hidden factors that contribute to weight gain, we can gain a deeper understanding of our bodies and how they respond to various stimuli. Armed with this knowledge, we can develop a holistic approach to weight management that addresses not just diet and exercise, but also the underlying factors that may be holding us back. With a focus on science-backed strategies, practical advice, and inspiring success stories, we can empower ourselves to take control of our health and achieve lasting weight loss. By shedding light on the hidden factors that contribute to weight gain, we can pave the way for a healthier, happier future.

Chapter 10
Start Your Transformation Today: Say Goodbye to

Frustration and Hello to a Healthier, Happier You

Are you tired of feeling stuck in a cycle of frustration when it comes to your health and weight? Have you tried countless diets and exercise plans only to see minimal results, if any at all? It's time to break free from the myths and misconceptions surrounding obesity and weight loss. In this chapter, we will delve into the real secrets to shedding pounds and achieving a healthier, happier you. Let's start by debunking the biggest myths about obesity that may have been holding you back. It's time to let go of the idea that quick fixes and extreme measures are the key to sustainable weight loss. Instead, we will explore effective and science-backed techniques that will not only help you shed pounds but also maintain a healthy lifestyle in the long run. One of the most important aspects to understand is that weight management is not just about what you eat or how much you exercise. Factors such as metabolism, hormones, and genetics play crucial roles in determining your body's ability to lose weight. By gaining insight into these factors, you can tailor your approach to weight loss to suit your unique needs and challenges. Creating a personalized plan that fits your lifestyle is essential for long-term success. This plan should not only focus on what you eat and how you move but also consider your emotional well-being and overall health. Sustainable weight loss is about making sustainable changes that you can maintain for life, rather than following a temporary solution that leaves you feeling frustrated and defeated. By taking the time to understand the truth behind obesity and weight loss, you can empower yourself to take control of your health and transform your life for the better. Say goodbye to the cycle of frustration and hello to a healthier, happier you. It's time to start your transformation today and embrace the journey towards a better version of yourself.

www.ingramcontent.com/pod-product-compliance
Lightning Source LLC
Chambersburg PA
CBHW072345270726
48659CB00023B/2389